HOW TO SOLVE MIGRAINE AND OTHER HEADACHES

What are the Triggers and How to Relief the Tension

By

Frank Woodworth

First Printing: 2019

Copyright © 2019 by Frank Woodworth

All rights reserved.

Printed in the United States

All rights reserved. This book or any of its parts may not be reproduced or used in any manner whatsoever without the express written permission of the author and publisher. However, brief quotations in an book review or scholarly journal are permitted.

Authors and their publications mentioned in this work and bibliography have their copyright protection. All brand and product names used in this book are trademarks, registered trademarks, or trade names and belong to the respective owners.

The author is unassociated with any product or vendor in this book.

DISCLAIMER

This book is for informational purposes only.

We assume no responsibility for what you do with the information contained in this book.

If you like what you learn in this book, a review would be MUCH appreciated! You can leave your REVIEW on the amazon site where you bought it.
Leaving reviews is the best way to help your fellow readers differentiate good books from terrible ones so make sure to help them out!

Contents

1. **CHAPTER ONE INTRODUCTION** 9
   - INTERNATIONAL CLASSIFICATION OF HEADACHE DISORDERS (ICHD) 10

2. **CHAPTER TWO TENSION TYPE HEADACHES (TTH)** 12
   - WHAT IS TTH AND WHAT ARE ITS SYMPTOMS? 12
   - WHAT CAUSES TENSION TYPE HEADACHES? 13
   - INTRODUCTION TO MIGRAINES 14
   - CAUSES OF MIGRAINES 15
   - CHANGE YOUR DIET 17
   - OVER-THE-COUNTER (OTC) RELIEF 19
   - PHYSICAL TREATMENTS 21

3. **CHAPTER THREE CLUSTER HEADACHES** 23
   - OTHER PRIMARY HEADACHES 24
   - HEMICRANIA CONTINUA 24
   - NEW DAILY PERSISTENT HEADACHE 25
   - THE MEDICAL RESPONSES TO HEADACHES 27

4. **CHAPTER FOUR MEDICAL TREATMENTS FOR TENSION TYPE HEADACHES** 28
   - AMITRIPTYLINE 28
   - MIRTAZAPINE 29
   - IBUPROFEN 30
   - NAPROXEN 30
   - INDOMETHACIN 31
   - KETOROLAC 31

5   CHAPTER FIVE MEDICAL TREATMENT FOR MIGRAINE 32

- SUMATRIPTAN 32
- BOTULINUM TOXIN 32
- PROPRANOLOL 33
- PIZOTIFEN 33
- ASPIRIN 34
- ERGOTAMINE 34

6   CHAPTER SIX MIGRAINE AND DAILY LIFESTYLE 35

- HOW TO PREVENT MIGRAINE OR HEADACHE ATTACKS: 36
- POOR SLEEP HABITS 36
- MEDICATION OVERUSE HEADACHE. 38
- JAW CLENCHING OR GRINDING 39
- MIGRAINE AND BAROMETRIC PRESSURE CHANGES: 40

7   CHAPTER SEVEN IDENTIFY THE CAUSE OF MIGRAINE 41

- TAKING THE FIRST STEPS 41
- IS GLUTEN YOUR PROBLEM? 46

8   CHAPTER EIGHT BEHAVIORAL CHANGES TO REDUCE HEADACHES 50

- COGNITIVE BEHAVIORAL THERAPY 53
- RELAXATION THERAPY 55
- BIOFEEDBACK THERAPY 58
- HOW CAN YOU AVOID THE WEATHER? 59
- BE CAREFUL HOW YOU WASH YOUR HAIR! 60

9   CHAPTER NINE DIFFERENT THERAPIES TO CURE HEADACHE 62

- HYPNOTHERAPY 62
- ACUPUNCTURE OR ACUPRESSURE 66
- MASSAGE THERAPY FOR HEADACHES… 70

OTHER NATURAL SOLUTIONS FOR HEADACHES 71
10 CHAPTER TEN HERBAL REMEDIES 73
    CONCLUSION 76
    REFERENCES 78

Acknowledgments

The author would like to acknowledge the assistance of Chris Payne, who helped him to accomplish this book. The author thanks him for all the contact moments where he patiently improved the author's work to create this book. Without his help, the author wouldn't be gotten so far to publish this book by now and found myself still in the editing state.

About the Author

Frank Woodworth had a good history of intense migraines. Sometimes it happens in the morning, and he had to call his boss of work to call in sick. Sometimes it happens during the day at work, which made it harder to call in sick.
Because no one can see that you experience a Migraine attack. And it gets even harder if you ask a colleague to bring you home because of your blurred vision.
You don't want to be a danger in traffic.

A migraine for Frank means:
1. Blurred vision on the left or right of his field of view.
2. Severe pain in his eyes or head, and sensitive to light.
3. Feeling the need of throwing up.
When going direct into bed, he won't experience the full attack or throwing up. And feeling sick afterward.

With the writing of his eBook, he put a stop to this pain with many solutions that this book provides. It is his wish, that you might find a solution in this book to get you rid of your migraine or headache. For him, the change in eating habits helped him to live headache free. A healthy lifestyle with sport and superfoods was his solution.

What will be yours?

1 Chapter One
INTRODUCTION

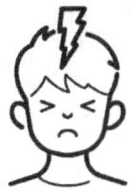

If you make a list of most common health complaints, you can never miss 'Headaches" from this list. Everyone knows what a headache is. It means 'pain in the head' and it is one of the few complaints which almost every person has made at least once in his life. Headache is quite variable in its attributes. Its impact can vary from distracting you from the daily routine to incapacitate you completely.

The headache affliction depends upon the cause of the headache. Mild and temporary headache directs the focus towards emotional distress or stress as a cause. Persistent and severe intensity headaches raise the doubt of notorious headaches like Migraine, Cluster headache or Tension headache as a cause. Headache along with any co-morbidity can lead to other causes like Hypertension or Brain cancer.

This e-book/book is designed to enable you in differentiating between the dangerous causes and non-dangerous causes of headaches. This will help you in making a decision when you should go for the home remedy and when you should consult your doctor about the headache. You will also come to know different natural ways to manage the headache.

Along with the natural remedies, you will also learn about common medications that are currently in use for headaches. Effect of different actions, remedies, and medications on headache and some common myths about the headache as well.

The official classification for headaches is known as "International classification of headache disorders (ICHD)" and it is also recognized by the World Health Organization (WHO). We will rely on this system to move forward.[1]

International Classification of Headache Disorders (ICHD)

The ICHD classification is used by health professionals worldwide and it is the most updated classification on headaches. The first edition of ICHD was published in 1988 and the most recent edition is published in 2018. With the help of ICHD classification criteria, you will get a systematic approach towards headaches in your mind and it will help you in understanding as well

The ICHD has a hierarchy of classification which includes the following three categories with the gradient of more important to less important.

- Primary Headaches
- Secondary Headaches
- Other Headaches

The primary headaches need the main attention here. Primary headaches include the following four headaches:

- Migraine
- Tension-Type Headache (TTH)
- Cluster headache
- Other primary headaches

After these four primary headaches, there are 14 secondary headaches as well. Secondary headache means that these headaches are a by-product of some other body issue. These body issues include majorly:

- Body Trauma
- Deformity of vessels (Hemorrhage, Fistula, Aneurysm, infection of vessels)
- Increased Intracranial pressure
- Abuse of any drug/substance
- Systemic infections
- Low Oxygen or excess carbon dioxide in the body
- Psychiatric issue
- Headache due to disorder of any facial or cranial structure

The classification of primary headaches includes those headaches in which you are unable to find any primary cause. We will evaluate different causes, address different queries and look upon different symptoms of headaches in the next couple of units.

2 Chapter Two

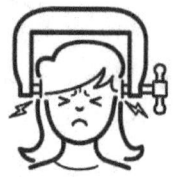

TENSION TYPE HEADACHES (TTH)

What is TTH and what are its symptoms?

TTH is the most common type of headache. It occurs in about 2/3rd of the general population. It can range from mild to severe headache incapacitating the quality of life of the patient [2].

TTH is divided into two subgroups:

- Infrequent Episodic TTH
- Frequent Episodic TTH
- Chronic TTH

Infrequent Episodic TTH includes one or fewer episodes per month. Frequent Episodic TTH includes more than one and less than 15 episodes per month for consecutive 3 months or more while Chronic TTH includes more than 15 episodes per month for consecutive 3 months or more.[3].

TTH is usually described as a band-like pain around the head. This pain is on both sides of the head. This pain is generally mild to moderate and daily routine physical activity has no role in aggravating it. The patient usually feels like his head is trapped between two objects on both sides of his head. TTH has no association with nausea and vomiting. Some studies have shown its association with tenderness (sensitivity to pain) and the association increases with an increase in the frequency of attacks.[3]

What causes tension-type headaches?

There was a famous hypothesis that TTH is caused by tension in the muscles of the scalp, head, and neck. Recently, research has proved this hypothesis wrong. The most common theory on the cause of TTH these days is that people who are more sensitive to pain tend to fall victim to TTH.[2].

Other possible triggers for TTH include the following:

- Dry eyes
- Flu
- Poor posture
- Alcohol
- Caffeine
- Eyestrain
- Emotional stress

These triggers are a few main causes of TTH. The triggers can extend too many other unique factors as well. So, you will hear about some patients having TTH with unique triggers as well. The best way to rule out unique triggers is to make a list of things, which you think are associated with the headache and rule out them one by one by inhibiting the triggers.

For example, there are many cases in which women suffer from tension-type headaches just before the start of their menstrual cycle. It may be a symptom of premenstrual syndrome as well. For some people, bright light flashes or loud noises can also cause a headache. So, the trigger for headaches can vary from person to person.

Introduction to Migraines

Migraine can produce throbbing pain or pulsating feeling usually on one side of the head. It usually has an association with nausea and vomiting. It's excruciating pain. Patients claim that there cannot be any pain worse than this one.

It seems to be that Migraine is gender-biased. 75% of migraine sufferers are women. Men are not exempted from this disease but its shown that women have more chances to get suffered from Migraines. This fact gave birth to the need for experiments to find out the relation between migraine and hormonal changes in women. Scientists have not yet succeeded to find any supporting evidence on this hypothesis.

Migraine symptoms include:

- Throbbing or pulsating pain
- Headache affecting just one side of the head
- Sound sensitivity (Phonophobia)
- Nausea
- Light sensitivity (Photophobia)

Usually, the average time for Migraine is between 4 to 72 hours but the pain can be shorter or longer than this period. As the routine activity makes the migraine worse, the patient is not able to do his routine activities until the migraine recedes.

About one-fifth migraine-sufferers have Aura. Aura is a warning sign before the pain of migraine starts. It usually lasts for 20 minutes. Now, what are these warning signs? Most commonly, Aura consists of visual symptoms such as blind spots, flashing lights or zigzag line resembling fort.

Aura can also consist of distorting figures, shapes. Some people have complained of difficulty in reading or driving as Aura of the migraine.

The source of these visual disturbances is not eyes. It comes from the brain. According to scientists, it is due to hyper-excitation of nerves in the brain that are activated before the migraine pain. [4]

Other symptoms of Aura include:

- Hearing noises
- Difficulty in speaking
- Pins and needles sensations in one arm or leg
- Uncontrollable jerking movement
- Weakness or pain in one side of the body

Causes of Migraines

No definitive cause of Migraine has been found yet. Research says that genetics and environmental factors seem to play an important role in migraine.

The trigeminal nerve is the nerve that has a major pain pathway. Migraine can be caused by changes in the brainstem and its interaction with the Trigeminal nerve. The balance of brain chemicals plays an important role in regulating the pain of the nervous system. Researchers have found that the serotonin (a brain chemical) levels drop during the Migraine attack. The drop in serotonin levels can lead to the release of neuropeptides by the Trigeminal nerve. These neuropeptides travel towards the outer covering of the brain and spinal cord (meninges) and result in migraine pain.

Other neurotransmitters such as Calcitonin gene-related peptide (CGRP) also have a role in the pain of Migraine.

Migraine triggers:

Migraine triggers include the following:

- Foods. Salty food, processed food or cheesy meal can trigger Migraines. Fasting or skipping meals can also trigger a migraine.

- Drinks. High caffeinated drinks, wines or alcohol can also trigger a migraine.

- Hormonal changes in women. Fluctuation in Estrogen seems to have an association with headaches. Many women complain of a headache just before or during the menstrual period when the estrogen level drops.

Some statistics show an increased tendency of migraine during pregnancy or menopause.
Hormone replacement therapies or oral contraceptives are also reported to worsen the headaches.

- Food additives. Food preservative Monosodium glutamate (MSG) or food sweetener Aspartame may trigger migraines in some people.

- Stress. Emotional or physical stress can also trigger a migraine.

- Medications. Vasodilators are claimed to worsen the migraine.

- Physical activity. Intense physical exertion, which also includes sexual activity, can also lead to migraines.

- Sensory stimuli. Sun glare, bright lights or any other strong visual stimulus can trigger a headache. Similarly, strong smells and loud sounds can also trigger a migraine.

- Change in environment. Change in weather can also lead to migraines. [5]

Knowledge of these triggering factors can help in identifying which one is your triggering factor and this can help in preventing the migraine.

You will learn many handy hacks in this unit to prevent or control migraines.

Change your Diet

As you have learned before, dietary triggers are very common factors in causing migraines. Sometimes, just making a simple change in your dietary routine can help you in getting rid of the migraine.

Water

Dehydration is not only known as a common trigger for migraines, it also causes many other disorders of the body. Drinking enough water can help you in preventing your migraine. What is the daily water need of a person?

According to WHO, a person should let his thirst decide the daily water rule. But average daily water intake for men should be 3.7 liters (15 cups) and average daily water intake for women should be 2.7 liters (12 cups). [6]

Caffeine

Caffeine is a very famous and strong chemical. It is the main component of coffee. Caffeine has a kind of dual role in the management of migraine.
If you are not a caffeine user and suffering from migraines, then you should try it as a remedy.
But if you are a caffeine-addicted person and suffering from migraine then decreasing caffeine intake can be beneficial.

Just to compare the pros and cons of caffeine, it is commonly used as a remedy in case of spinal headaches (headache after spinal anesthesia). So, it can be of different use in every person's case. But you should keep in mind caffeine as an option.

Monosodium Glutamate

Monosodium glutamate (MSG) is used as a flavor enhancer in many foods. It adds savory and salty taste to the food and is very commonly used in the food industry.

Mostly, people think that MSG is an ingredient of Chinese foods only. However, this is just a misconception, MSG is added to all types of processed foods available in your local supermarket.

MSG is commonly found in meat tenderizer, soya sauce, frozen dinners, gravies, soups, and many other foods. It is available under many different names as well so you must be careful and focus on 'MSG' when trying to identify it. [7]

Tension Type Headaches (TTH)

Commonly, people who eat more food in fast food restaurants (not only Chinese restaurants) than eating home-made foods are prone to the hazards of MSG. It is also a known trigger of migraines so better avoid it if you are suffering from headaches plus a fast-food addicted guy.

Over-the-Counter (OTC) Relief

Many conventional OTC medications are not very helpful in the management of migraine and researchers are still struggling with the answer. Besides the OTC medications, there are many other medications available in your local pharmacy that is very helpful.

Fish Oil

Fish oil has omega fatty acid series in it which acts as an anti-inflammatory drug, much similar to the role of NSAIDs and steroids but with much fewer side effects.
Fish oil decreases the inflammation and kills the inflammatory substances in the blood vessels, thus helping in decreasing pain.

You can get the fish oil either by eating fatty fishes like Salmon and Mackerel or by having fish oil capsules available in most pharmacies.

Peppermint Oil

For some migraine-sufferers, rubbing peppermint oil on the sides of their head or at the site of pain helps in reducing migraines. Of course, this is not suitable for everyone to do and is not a 100% remedy formula. But still, it helps in reducing the migraine.

Vitamin B2 (Riboflavin)

An oral dose of 400 mg of vitamin B2 daily can help in preventing migraines for some people. If 400 mg is not producing the result, you should consider adjusting your dose by consulting your physician. Usually, people who experience dark urination or who make a complaint of frequent urination need more vitamin B2.

Magnesium

Migraines that are associated with the menstrual cycle or Auras are claimed to be reduced with oral Magnesium intake. Try 400-600 mg of a daily dose of Magnesium.

But if you experience abdominal pain or diarrhea then try to lower the dosage.

CoEnzymeQ10 (CoQ10)

Though it is an expensive option, CoEnzymeQ10 is famous for reducing all types of headaches especially migraines. Try 300 mg oral daily dose for a week to see if it is useful to combat migraines, but if it's not useful, then do not continue it because it is an expensive option.

Ginger

For those who complain about nausea during a migraine, ginger can be the best remedy for it. It can be used in both raw and cooked forms. It can be taken as ginger ale or in capsule form.

One thing you need to make sure before using any ginger product is that the ingredients should not be artificial flavors but natural ginger. Some anecdotal evidence also supports than ginger can reduce migraine pain so ginger can be the right choice to treat migraine.

Butterbur

Butterbur is a plant usually found in Germany. It is also known as parasites. Large experimental evidence has supported the effectiveness of butterbur in the treatment of migraine.

Research also supports its use for nausea and asthma. The main issue is this remedy is not widely available in non-German areas so you may need to order it online.

Physical Treatments

Some physical options are also available for the management of migraine pain. While supplements and dietary changes are also available, physical actions are easy to use and often work quickly.

Sensory Deprivation

For some people, sensory deprivation is helpful to reduce the pain of migraines. Migraine sufferers are more sensitive to sound and light and exposure to any of these two stimuli can worsen the migraine.

One way to achieve sensory deprivation is lying down in a tub full of water. The temperature of the water should be normal. Turn off all the lights in the washroom and lie deep enough to cover your ear in the water. This will inhibit most of the sensory input to disturb you and thus will help you in minimizing the pain of migraines.

Compresses

This is the oldest method used for the management of the migraine. Many people have also claimed it to be the quickest method to eliminate migraines. Basically, in this method, you are supposed to compress your head by tying something around it.

You simply tie a band tightly around your head. It numbs the sensations of migraines and helps you get rid of migraines quickly.

Ice Bands

Putting ice bands around the head is also a very effective method. You need to put Ice in plastic bags, gently wrap the plastic bags in a towel and then wrap the towel around your head. Another easy way is to buy Ice bands designed specifically for migraines.

Similarly, there are heat pads available in the market. You just need to fill it with hot water, close the lid and compress it against your head multiple times.

3 Chapter Three
CLUSTER HEADACHES

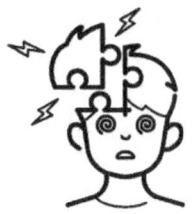

Cluster headaches are named so because people who suffered from this type of headache complain of many headaches in the form of a 'cluster' which usually has a little relaxation period between them. Cluster headaches cause severe discomfort and its duration can vary between 15 minutes to 3 hours.

The onset of a cluster headache is very quick and without any Aura. Its intensity is severe and it is usually unilateral which means it only causes pain to one side of the head. Some doctors also name it as 'shifting headache' because it shifts the direction in every attack.

Cluster headaches are also gendered biased and it is men who are more inclined to have cluster headaches. A feeling of discomfort or a slight one-sided burning is the warning signs a person can have before a cluster headache. When the cluster headache starts, the pain may spread to jaw, neck, ear and other parts of the head. [8]

The main reason for the cluster headache is still not revealed. Many people misunderstand this pain as indications of brain cancer or multiple sclerosis until they consult the doctor.

The sufferers of this headache claim it as the worst pain ever. Many women who have cluster headache consider it as painful as childbirth without an epidural. Usually, people feel the pain behind the eyes or temple or on the sides of their head and sometimes it radiates to the neck as well. Cluster headache sufferers consider this pain like the pain of gunshot in the face. [9]

The cluster headache attacks the sufferer's at-least three to four times a day for many weeks. One cannot guess the pain of such a patient in its full meaning. It truly incapacitates the person to perform its daily routine work.

It was Dr.B.T Horton who first coined the concept of Cluster headache and propagated it in 1939. Cluster headache is also known as "suicide headache". Because it pushes the sufferer to commit suicide. [10]

Luckily, almost 3 out of 1000 people suffer from the cluster headache.
This makes this type of headache pretty rare. But those who suffer from Cluster headache claims it as the worst pain they have ever felt.

Trigeminal neuralgia is a chronic pain that affects the trigeminal nerve which carries sensation to the face. That way the trigeminal neuralgia is felt in the area of cheek instead of eyes or temple.

Other primary headaches

Many different headaches are also primary headaches categorized as primary because there is no primary cause or medical association is found in these headaches. These headaches include:

1- Hemicrania continua
2- New daily persistent headache

Hemicrania continua

It's a persistent one-sided headache that is usually continuous. The IHS system of classification for Hemicrania continua states that for the proper diagnosing of this headache, a sufferer has to suffer from this headache for at least three months while also showing these symptoms:

- There must be non-shifting persistent pain on one side of the head (unilateral).

- Most of the time, the pain should be moderate in intensity. Though, periods with severe intensity pain can also be there.

- The pain should be continuous without any remission and without omitting any day.

A Hemicrania continuum is not limited to headaches only. It also includes nose and eyes related symptoms such as nasal congestion or crying. This feature differentiates it from other primary headaches.

There are a few exceptions where all the symptoms of Hemicrania are as per literature but remission is also present. Doctors diagnose such cases as Hemicrania because they fulfill all the other requirements of Hemicrania continua.

New daily persistent headache

This condition is recently included in the second edition of ICHD in 2004 by the International Headache Society (IHS). It is included in the major group of primary headaches. According to the criteria of ICHD, the daily persistent headache include the following symptoms:

- The history of headache should be at least 3 months long.
- The pain must be unremitting and continuous.
- The pain must have the following four features:

  - The pain must be mild to moderate.
  - The pain must be on both sides of the head.
  - The pain should not aggravate by routine physical activity like climbing the stairs or walking.
  - The pain must be tightening or pressing in nature. The patient should not complain of throbbing nature.

- Vomiting or nausea should not accompany the headache.
- The patient should not be sensitive to light or noise.

This condition is usually difficult to diagnose because it has the characteristics of both migraine and tension-type headache. Clinicians usually misdiagnose this condition.

There is also an alarming alert associated with this condition. Patients who suffer from spontaneous brain fluid (cerebrospinal fluid) leak also mimic kind of similar symptoms. So, whenever you feel or see such symptoms, it is better to consult a doctor so that he can run a few imaging tests such as MRI to rule out another dangerous differential diagnosis.

Moreover, doctors may also need to do a bacterial culture test by doing lumbar puncture to rule out infection before making the diagnosis of a daily persistent headache.

The medical responses to headaches

Describing all the symptoms of headaches in detail makes it clear that these conditions are not going away without treatment. People usually go for natural remedies at first, which we have discussed in a very detailed manner.

Those who are not getting good results with natural remedies need to seek medical attention. Still, people with mild symptoms first try the over-the-counter painkillers to get rid of the headaches. But those who are suffering from severe symptoms go to seek medical consultation.

In the next units, we are going to have a detailed discussion about the medical treatment options for headaches and insight about the side effects of those drugs.

4 Chapter Four

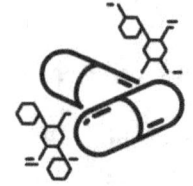

MEDICAL TREATMENTS FOR TENSION TYPE HEADACHES

If you only get an occasional headache then most likely you are suffering from an episodic tension-type headache.

In this case, people usually go for over-the-counter painkillers. Common people are not aware of the side effects of these drugs. The side effects can be a potential threat to the patient.

For chronic tension-type headaches, there are also several options available. Following are some of the most common options:

Amitriptyline

Amitriptyline is a prototype drug of the tricyclic antidepressant family. This drug is in use for four decades now. This drug has anxiolytic and sedative properties.

This drug is mainly indicated in the prophylaxis of the Migraine and the management of Tension headache.

Some of the undesired documented side effects include constipation, blurred vision, dry mouth, weight gain, insomnia, and nausea. In severe cases and overdose, this drug can cause arrhythmia, depression, hypotension, depression, and psychosis.

Mirtazapine

Mirtazapine is an alpha-2 antagonist drug which means it helps in increasing neurotransmission. This drug is mainly used as an anti-depressant but it is also found to be effective in the management of chronic tension-type headache and migraine.

Unfortunately, this drug has a long list of side effects. The common side-effects include weight gain, dizziness, blurred vision, restless leg syndrome or shallow breathing.

Some other side-effects, which occur due to overdose, include convulsion, sexual dysfunction, and anxiety.

Paracetamol

Paracetamol is an antipyretic and analgesic agent. Paracetamol is an important drug used for the treatment of mild to moderate pain in conditions where the anti-inflammatory effect is not required. This drug has better efficacy and fewer side-effects than aspirin.

This drug is mainly indicated in tension headaches, fever and mild to moderate pain.

Paracetamol, though commonly used, also have overdose side-effects. The adverse side-effects include blood disorders, liver damage, and bronchospasm. The signs and symptoms of acute over-dosage include liver failure, kidney failure, and hypoglycemic coma.

Ibuprofen

Ibuprofen also belongs to an NSAID family. Antipyretic and analgesic are its main features. This drug is equal to Paracetamol or aspirin in its anti-inflammatory effect but it is better analgesic than Paracetamol or aspirin. This drug is also available for both oral and topical usage.

This drug is effective in tension headache, mild to moderate pain, musculoskeletal pain, and migraines.

People with hypertension, bronchospasm, gastric or kidney disorders are not recommended to go for ibuprofen.

The side effects include hypertension, low platelet count, peptic ulcer, gastric pain or blood in vomitus as well. The signs and symptoms after acute over-dosage include cardiac arrhythmia, seizure, kidney failure or liver failure.

Naproxen

Naproxen is also famous for its antipyretic and analgesic effects. This drug was approved by the FDA in 1976. It is superior to many other drugs in the treatment of migraine and tension headaches.

Primary indications of Naproxen include tension headache, Migraine, and musculoskeletal pain.

The side effects of Naproxen include Hepatitis, Anemia, damage of kidneys and damage to the liver. It can also cause gastric ulcers.

The signs and symptoms after acute over-dosage include vomiting, seizure, nausea, hearing loss, and hypertension.

Indomethacin

Indomethacin belongs to the NSAID family. It relieves pain and fever. This drug is more toxic but more effective than aspirin. Indomethacin is not primarily made for headache but in certain cases, headache pain seems to respond to Indomethacin and you need to consult your doctor for using this drug for headache. This drug is administered orally.

Its side-effects include an increase in blood Potassium level, a decrease in platelets and white blood cells, hepatitis, and GI bleeding.

Acute over-dosage includes vomiting, dizziness, convulsion, numbness, and mental confusion.

Ketorolac

Ketorolac is a drug that can be given on trial for resistant tension-type headaches. Do consult with your doctor before using it.

5 Chapter Five
MEDICAL TREATMENT FOR MIGRAINE

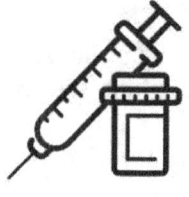

Though, most drugs that are discussed for tension-type headache can also be given to Migraine sufferers. Migraine pain is throbbing in nature and it is usually on one side of the head.

Sumatriptan

Sumatriptan is a 5-HT 1 agonist. This drug can be given orally or via intravenous injection. This drug is very much effective in the management of acute migraine attacks. It reduces the dilatation of blood vessels which is associated with a throbbing headache. Thus, it reduces the pain of migraines.

Sumatriptan is not an effective drug for prophylaxis of migraine. This drug is indicated in conditions like acute migraine attack, cluster headaches or migraine.

The irreversible side-effects of Sumatriptan include cardiac arrhythmia, bradycardia, tachycardia, angina, ventricular fibrillation or atrioventricular block. Sumatriptan can also lead to myocardial infarction.

Botulinum toxin

Scalp injection of botulinum toxin type A (BT-A) can help in the management of migraine headaches. Clinical trials have shown that a single botulinum toxin prevents the migraine attacks for 3 months.

Botulinum toxin is claimed to have an extended analgesic effect and it is not related to skeletal muscle relaxation. The effect of BT-A stays for 8 to 12 weeks and then again the pain of migraine will start so actually you need to have repeated BT-A injections to maintain its analgesic effect.

BT-A is usually not harmful to the brain because it does not cross the blood-brain barrier [12].

Propranolol

Propranolol is an anti-anginal, anti-hypertensive and anti-arrhythmic agent. It can be administered intravenously or orally and it can be used in the prevention of anxiety disorders and migraines.

Propranolol is primarily indicated for hypertension and cardiac issues but it is very famous for its role in preventing migraines. It is also useful in reducing raised intracranial pressure.

The irreversible side-effects of propranolol include visual hallucinations, decreased platelets, and low blood glucose levels. Acute over-dosage of propranolol causes convulsions, coma, and seizure.

Pizotifen

Pizotifen is used for the prevention of migraine. It is indicated in the prophylaxis of vascular headache or migraine prophylaxis.

The side-effects of pizotifen include dry mouth, dizziness, increased appetite, and drowsiness.

Aspirin

Similar to Paracetamol and naproxen, aspirin is a famous over-the-counter drug and it also belongs to the NSAID family. This drug has anti-thrombin, analgesic, antipyretic and anti-inflammatory effects.

Besides the cardiac and brain indications, this drug indicates migraine.

The side-effects include rhinitis, hepatitis, hepatomegaly, gastrointestinal bleeding, and edema.

The acute overdose of aspirin can lead to hyperglycemia, kidney failure, liver failure, and vertigo.

Ergotamine

It is an alkaloid derived from ergot. Ergotamine is commonly used as a painkiller in the treatment of cluster headaches and migraines.

It is indicated in conditions like vascular headache, migraine and prophylactic treatment of vascular headache.

The irreversible side-effects include fibrillation of the heart, lung cavity, abdominal cavity, and stroke.

The signs and symptoms after acute overdosage include tachycardia, nausea, vomiting, diarrhea, and cold extremities

6 Chapter Six

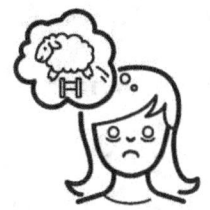

MIGRAINE AND DAILY LIFESTYLE

Most of the migraine sufferers complain that they usually have migraine attacks from 4 am to 9 am. Migraine headache is the most common pain that every person suffers at least once in his life. Some main reasons are mentioned below that may awake you from sleep:

- Insomnia
- Stress
- Medication overuse headache
- Hormones
- Allergens
- Intracranial hypotension
- Sleep apnea
- Low blood sugar level
- Jaw clenching or grinding

How to prevent migraine or headache attacks:

- Stay hydrated
- Do not clench your jaw
- Avoid stress
- Develop good sleep habits
- Maintain blood sugar level
- Identify the allergens which trigger the migraine and avoid them

Poor Sleep Habits

Poor sleeping habit is the most frequent migraine trigger. During sleeping, the brain performs many restorative functions, which affect different parts of the human body.

Neurotransmitters are chemical messengers. They send information between neurons via a synapse. A sleep-deprived person does not provide enough time for such restorative functions does cause a headache.

Insufficient sleep can also cause a physical and emotional type of pain. Peaceful sleep minimizes the chances of migraines. There are a few reasons that cause migraine when you wake up in the morning:

- Disturbed sleep
- Too little sleep
- Poor quality sleep
- The dramatic shift in sleep routine i.e. jetlag
- Too much sleep
- Irregular sleep routines

According to the studies on the people having a migraine, people who have migraines also have complications while sleeping. They also state that insufficient sleep is the primary trigger of headaches for them.

SLEEP DISORDERS

SLEEP APNEA

It is a type of disorder that disturbs the pattern of breathing when a person is sleeping. Sleep apnea usually disturbs the quality of sleep. That is the reason the person feels sleepy and tired the whole day.

Almost 80% of sleep apnea sufferers do not know that they are suffering from it. Commonly their partner let them know about this disorder.

Scientists are still struggling to find any solid association of migraine and sleep apnea. The primary reason that pushes a person toward sleep apnea is snoring. It is considered as the warning sign of sleep apnea.

INSOMNIA

Insomnia is one of the major sleep issues in which is present in many migraine sufferers. They also have other symptoms like

1-Difficult to fall asleep.
2-Wake up too early in the morning
3-Wake up in the night and face difficulty to sleep again
4-Feel sleepy upon waking.

There are two types of insomnia

1-Primary insomnia
2-Acute insomnia

Primary insomnia:

In this type of insomnia, a person usually has sleeping problems but these problems are not directly associated with other medical conditions.

Secondary insomnia:

In this type of insomnia, a person's sleeping problems are directly associated with other medical condition such as:

- Heartburn
- Asthma
- Depression
- Gouty Arthritis [13]

MEDICATION OVERUSE HEADACHE.

Medication overuse headache is usually a type of headache which occurs when a person takes too many analgesics to relieve a headache. Usually, this type of headache occurs in those patients who are already suffering from tension headaches or migraine and they are taking medication for more than six months. Medication overuse headache is the third most common type of headache. It is notorious for its severe intensity and incapacitating nature. It is also commonly named as rebound headache.

Do Botox injections help eliminate migraines?

Though Botox injections have been discussed in the previous unit. It needs a little addition in this section as well. Botox injections are not a permanent solution for headaches. Usually, you start with sessions of Botox on many areas of your scalp and head and the results begin to appear after 2-3 sessions. Still, to maintain the effects, you need to repeat the Botox injections on regular intervals otherwise the effect will fade out.

SIDE EFFECTS

- Botox is used for migraines as treatment. But some people should try trial oral medication before choosing Botox as an option
- Botox causes weakness of muscle, vision problem, eyelids drooping and also affects the swallowing, speaking, and breathing process.
- The safety level of Botox for pregnant women and breastfeeding mothers is still a topic of debate. You should always consult your doctor before booking an appointment of Botox

Jaw clenching or grinding

Jaw clenching is a habit of clenching your jaws. People do not usually realize about jaw clenching and they even clench their jaws during sleep. This habit leads to stiffness in jaw muscles, pain in the temporal region and even damaging to teeth. You should try to work out ways to break this behavior because this can lead to headaches disturbing your daily routine.

Migraine and barometric pressure changes:

The storms, high temperature, and humidity in the air can triggers migraine because when there is a change in pressure due to weather, they trigger the electrical and chemical changes in the brain which annoy the nerves and result in headache.

If you want to prevent migraines in these situations, just use the weather forecast to predict when you have a migraine and take some medicine one or two days before storms.

7 Chapter Seven

IDENTIFY THE CAUSE OF MIGRAINE

Taking the first steps...

If you want to live your life merrily and get rid of headaches in a natural way without medicines, the best way is that you identify the cause that triggers a migraine. It is not easy to identify the root cause of headaches for headache sufferer but sometimes it is a very common factor that triggers the migraine in a person.

To get rid of headaches, there is a very basic step you need to follow. Develop a habit to write a journal or diary about your migraine. If you get to know the triggering factors of your migraine then avoiding those factors is better than any medication for your headache. Many causes trigger a migraine-like:

- Poor diet
- Insufficient sleep
- Environmental factors
- Food
- Stress
- Drinks

Usually, the cause of migraine differs from person to person. Only a migraine-sufferer can identify the triggering factor of his migraine.

How To Solve Migraine And Other Headaches

For some people, it is very easy to find out the cause of their migraines. But most often, figuring out the triggering factor is one of the toughest jobs in the world. If you feel that you are stuck in a similar situation then pick a diary and jot down all the activities relevant to migraines. Ruling out every suspected factor is your way to find out the cause of migraines. Some example of suspected factors includes but not limited to:

- How much do you sleep?
- What do you eat and drink?
- When do you eat and drink?
- Where are you (at home, at the office or on vacation)?
- Have you done the exercise on that day or not?
- Have periods or not (for females)?
- What were you doing at that time when the migraine started?
- Which medicine do you take and in what dosage?
- What was the intensity of migraines?
- What was the weather at that time?

You can rate the intensity of your migraine in the migraine diary. By using a scale of 1 to 5 level, 1 denoting to a no migraine day and 5 when you have a severe level of migraine pain. Keep this record in a workable way so that you can easily find the root cause of the migraine. The main effort in this whole process is to figure out the reason that triggers the migraine.

There will be some possibility that you may not have a migraine, maybe it is any other type of headaches like a tension headache or cluster headache.

IDENTIFY THE CAUSE OF MIGRAINE

To diagnose which type of headache you have, you should consult a doctor or read the previous chapters of this book.

Tension headache includes throbbing pain in one or both sides of the head. The main cause of this headache is stress and continuous work like having a hectic working day. The causes of tension-type headaches are already discussed in the previous chapters of this book. You may have tension headaches if your headache type and other symptoms are similar to them.

It is a fact that causes of headaches vary from person to person. Food is also a very prominent example of this. Certain foods can be incompatible with the internal chemistry of certain people leading to any type of headache while similar foods can be pretty much normal and non-stimulating for others.

Keep a record that what you eat in your every meal so that you can easily find what you eat before the beginning of a migraine attack. It is a promising step to figure out the triggering thing.

According to studies, the time gap between the onset of headache and triggering factors can vary from the range of minutes to days. Every headache-sufferer has its time gap.

In some unusual cases, people do not have a headache for a few days after the occurrence of a trigger. A headache usually begins 3 to 12 hours after a trigger. However, you should observe your migraine diary for a few days before considering anything as a trigger.

How To Solve Migraine And Other Headaches

The purpose of writing all the activities before and after the headache attack is to identify the thing that triggers the headache. Maybe it is one or more triggers that cause a headache.

If you are succeeded in identifying the cause that triggers your headache, then you can limit the use of triggering factors or even eliminate it from your life.

Now if you find out the specific food or the specific stressful event that triggers your headache then your priority should be to avoid that trigger or event.

It is not practical to avoid everything that triggers headaches for you. For example, if you have identified that tension of office work is the triggering factor of your headache, then you can at least try to minimize or kill the tension. If you are not able to reduce the tension to a sufficient level then maybe quitting the job is an only viable option for you.

However, identifying the main cause that triggers your headache is a great victory. After knowing the cause, you can take steps to reduce or eliminate it. For example, considering the previous scenario, if the office stress triggers the headache then you can organize your work habit by including some gaps for relaxation in between the work hours. Relaxing exercises slow down your heart rate and lower your blood pressure. There are many types of techniques for relaxation.

IDENTIFY THE CAUSE OF MIGRAINE

Some of them are as follows:

- Meditation
- Yoga
- Deep breathing
- Massage
- Aromatherapy
- Music and art therapy

For relaxation, some people engage themselves in different activities like:

- Gardening
- Painting
- Reading a book
- Listening to music
- Solving any puzzle
- Other hobbies

You can try some yoga techniques to relieve stress and anxiety. Yoga is the combination of physical postures; deep breathing and meditation, which help to get you, relax. It will increase your work efficiency.

But sometimes, it is not possible to stay away from the thing that triggers headaches in your life until and unless you identify it. You just want to learn how to deal with that trigger successfully and prevent headaches for the next time.

It is usually claimed that limiting your caffeine and alcohol intake can decrease the intensity of migraines. One should also avoid using both beverages on the same day.

How To Solve Migraine And Other Headaches

There are many different types of migraine or tension headaches which are pretty common. Some of them are as follows:

- Headache with rhinitis (hay fever).
- Allergic reactions due to food or beverages like soya-bean, wheat, egg milk or peanut.
- Flashy lights.
- High volume noise.
- Specific fragrances or smells.
- Smoke can also cause migraine and tension headache

By writing a migraine diary, you find the cause that triggers your headache and then you try to eliminate it from your life with maximum effort.

If in case, you are still unable to find out the trigger for your headache, I just want to let you that it is not the end of the world. In the next units, you are going to find more solutions for your headache.

Is Gluten your problem?

Gluten is a protein that you can find in several grain foods like wheat, spelled, barley and rye. Wheat is the most commonly consumed grain. Therefore, gluten is the major

part of the bread and most of the other carbohydrates. But there is some gluten-free grain like oats, corn, rice, and millet.

IDENTIFY THE CAUSE OF MIGRAINE

A few people suffer from a disease called Celiac disease, a disease in which the immune system produces antibodies against the gluten that is an integral part of wheat. This decreases gluten digestion markedly leading to poor health.

Symptoms of celiac disease are as follows:

- Diarrhea
- Blotting
- Weight loss
- Instant fall in health line

If you have all of the above symptoms then you need to cut down the items containing gluten from your diet like:

- Wheat
- Soy sauce
- Semolina
- Rye
- Bulgur
- Spelled
- Durum

After the research of many years, medical science has proven that there is some connection between migraine and gluten. So, if you are a regular migraine sufferer then you may also have a problem in digesting the gluten. By avoiding the gluten item you can lessen the chances of having a migraine. There is much gluten-free grain which

you can add after removing the gluten item from your diet like:
- vegetables, including starchy vegetables like potatoes, peas, and corn
- fruits
- lentils
- quinoa
- buckwheat
- rice
- tapioca
- most of the dairy products
- meat and poultry (if prepared without frying and bread)
- beans[13]

The scientist has claimed that celiac disease can result in inflammation of the central nervous system. This was relieved in a study in which MRI brain reports of celiac disease sufferers were compared with that of non-sufferers. This inflammation of CNS has been found in indirect relation with migraines. Eliminating the gluten product from your diet can regress these changes and can help in curing the migraine.[14]

According to Mario Giacovazzo, migraine sufferers are at high risk of developing the celiac disease as well. His study claims that the risk is 10 times greater. Here you can appreciate the link between these two diseases and the fact any of them can lead to the development of another disease. [15]

In another research, Isabel Camino state that the gluten-free diet improves the blood flow to the brain. By having gluten

IDENTIFY THE CAUSE OF MIGRAINE

free diet, it may be possible that the migraine ends completely or reduce the intensity and duration of migraine.

All the researches about gluten and migraine show that there is a visible connection between both of these diseases. So by having a Gluten-free diet you can get rid of or minimize the intensity and duration of the migraine completely. It also boosts the blood circulation towards the brain helping the brain to get rid of toxic substances and in getting access to fresh nutrients thus minimizing the severity of migraine.

8 Chapter Eight
BEHAVIORAL CHANGES TO REDUCE HEADACHES

As already mentioned, if you know what triggers your headache, you can easily end or lessen the pain of a headache. You may have multiple causes of your headache. For this, keep a diary and a journal in which you maintain your all record of your daily activities, through which you can find out all possible reason that triggers a migraine.

Even so, many doctors believe that if a person changes his lifestyle by avoiding the causes that lead to headaches, he can end or reduce the intensity and duration of the headache.

If it is difficult to pinpoint the cause of a migraine or chronic headaches, you can make the following changes and check their effectiveness.

Many doctors believe that if a person starts doing 20 to 30 minutes of cardio exercise a day, it will help to reduce the intensity of migraines.

Daily exercise boosts the circulation of blood in our body. It may not have any direct effects that stop or eliminate the headache, but it will help to minimize the intensity and occurrence of headaches for sure.

For instance, if a person is having tension headaches due to stress, the optimal way to reduce stress is exercise. According to the research, the cardio exercise is found helpful in letting the negative feelings and emotions out of the body such as anger, stress or frustration. As these emotions are one of the major causes of tension headache, it has a direct impact in decreasing the frequency of headache.

According to the research, there is a great possibility to stop or reduce the headache if you just walk for 20 minutes once a day. There are several sports that you can do instead of walk like:

- Hiking
- Tennis
- Swimming
- Cycling
- Jumping rope
- Brisk walk
- Jogging

And many more it depends on your choice of what you like to do. Most of the people also like to do yoga and Pilates. [16]

Most of the doctors recommend their patients to have a regular sleep pattern for 8 hours. Now a day, people cannot have sufficient sleep due to the overuse of social media. Now it is proven that there is a biological link between insufficient sleep and headache.

If you have a migraine or chronic headache, sleeping is the best option to get relieved from the severe headache pain. Until and unless the pain is unbearable and you are unable to sleep then it is not good enough for you.
Diet also plays an important role in eliminating the headache from your life. The common triggers that cause headaches are foods containing Tyramine such as:

How To Solve Migraine And Other Headaches

- Smoked fish
- Aged cheese
- Figs
- Red wine
- Chocolate
- Nuts
- Bananas
- Peanut butter
- Dairy products

According to medical experts, aspartame can also trigger a headache in some people but it is not proven yet.

MSG can be included in the list of most common triggers for migraine and chronic headache. It is observed that a person who uses monosodium glutamate has far more chances of having a migraine and chronic headaches than a person who is given a placebo.

You can also try to reduce migraine and chronic pain by smashing the routine cycle. Many people claim that they have experienced a certain pattern that becomes predictable by the time. When you can predict the cycle of migraine or chronic pain, you can simply smash it and lessen the pain of migraine or chronic headache.

When you find out the cause of your headache you can avoid that triggering thing physically or sometimes mentally. It will help you to stop or reduce migraine and tension headaches. If you follow this routine, you can remove the migraine and chronic headache in the future.

When you think you are feeling stress and frustration, try to take deep breaths that will make you feel better. Try auto-hypnosis or visualization, it will refresh your mind.

BEHAVIOURAL CHANGES TO REDUCE HEADACHES

In auto-hypnosis or visualization, you visualize something that you love to do. It may be a scene in which you are playing games or in which you are beating the villains, anything that you love to do. This visualization will dictate your mind that you are in a very enjoyable environment right now. The mind will release serotonin in a reaction that elevates your mood and help you in combating the stress.

Some people have claimed that these visualization techniques are very effective for them. Both of these therapies reduce the intensity of migraines and chronic headaches. The best thing about this practice is that it has no side-effects on your brain and body.

Some of the behavioral changes have already been discussed in the previous units. But still, there are many other therapies like [17]

- Cognitive-behavioral therapy
- Relaxation therapy
- Biofeedback therapy

Cognitive-behavioral therapy

It is a type of behavioral therapy, which is mainly used to cure depression and anxiety. It is also useful for other mental disorders. In this therapy, your feelings, thoughts, actions, and sensations are associated and all your adverse feeling confine you. There is a hypothesis that the thoughts, feelings, and actions of a human being are interconnected. Cognitive-behavioral therapy is based on this hypothesis.

Cognitive-behavioral therapy breaks huge problems into smaller ones. With the help of logic, it helps to change your mentality about negative thoughts and make you feel better.

In CBT, they deal with your current problems. They do not have any concern with your past.

Cognitive-behavioral therapy can be used in:

- Phobias
- Sleeping disorder
- Problems of alcohol misuse
- Eating disorders like bulimia and anorexia
- Panic disorder
- Obsessive-compulsive disorder(OCD)
- Post-traumatic stress disorder(PTSD)

It is also used sometimes to heal long term health conditions like:

- Chronic fatigue syndrome
- Irritable bowel syndrome

The session of CBT is usually 5 to 20 minutes long. The sessions are held every week or every fortnight. In these sessions, the experts get to know about your weakness or your phobias and change that phobia into good thoughts with the help of logic.

Some of the common advantages of CBT are:

- It gives the best result if you try it along with medications.
- As compared to other talking therapies, this therapy takes less time.
- It is a very useful practice that you can continue even after the treatment ends.

Some of the disadvantages are:

- This treatment is not for the persons having complex mental conditions.
- In this treatment, most of the work is done by you. If you do not follow the therapist's recommendation then all of these sessions are in vain. [18]

Relaxation therapy

Relaxation therapy is a type of therapy that not only relaxes your mind but also relaxes the body from tension and stress. It is useful for your everyday stress and stress-related health care problems.

If you feel that you are in stress, try this therapy. It will lessen your stress. You do not need any special effort to learn these techniques.

The perks of relaxation therapy are as follows:

- You can do it at any place
- It is free of cost.
- And the best thing is that it has no side-effects on your brain and body.

Relaxation therapy:

- Regulates your heart rate.
- Improve digestion.
- Smooths you breathe rate.
- Improves the quality of sleep.
- Reduces the activity of stress hormones.
- Improves the blood flow to the major muscles.
- Reduces your anger and frustration.
- It improves your power to solve any problems.
- Reduces chronic pain and muscle tension.
- It improves your mood and concentration.
- Controls your blood sugar level.

Types of relaxation therapy

Many health experts and psychotherapists recommend relaxation therapies to reduce stress and frustration. Many instructors teach these techniques but you can also learn it on your own. It helps you to focus on something calming and enhances the perception of your body.

The names of some relaxation therapies are:

- Autogenic relaxation
- Progressive muscles relaxation
- Visualization

Autogenic relaxation

Autogenic means are self-generated. A thing that is created from your inside. In this technique, body perception and visual imagery are used to reduce anxiety. You repeat some suggestions and words in your mind; it helps to reduce the tension from your mind and body.

For instance, you imagine a peaceful scene in which your heart rate is slowing down, breath is getting smooth and your muscles are relaxed.

Progressive muscles relaxation

Progressive muscle relaxation is a treatment in which your focus is on tensing and relaxing each muscle of your body. This therapy helps you to focus on tensing and relaxing muscles. After this, you will feel improvement in perceiving the sensations.

In this therapy, you can start from the muscles of your toes and then gradually move towards the muscles of the neck. First, you will tense and relax the muscles of your toes, then legs, then thighs, then back, then shoulder and eventually ending at the muscles of head and neck.
You can also go in the opposite direction. Tense each pair of muscles for 5 seconds and then take a break of 30 seconds, and do it again.

Visualization

Visualization is a type of therapy in which you imagine the desired image in your mind to enjoy a peaceful and happy trip to your desired place.

There are associations of many senses in this therapy. For this, you have to sit in a quiet area, wear loose clothes, close your eyes and breathe deeply. Now you aim to focus and think positively.

For example, imagine that you are on the beach and you are feeling the breezy air, the sound of rushing waves and the heat of sunlight on your body.

There are many other types of relaxation techniques like:

- Yoga
- Tai chi
- Hydrotherapy
- Aromatherapy
- Biofeedback
- Meditation
- Deep breathing
- Music and Art therapy
- Massage [19]

Biofeedback therapy

Biofeedback therapy is a type of therapy that helps a person to gain more control over the involuntary action functions. It is mainly used to treat chronic headaches, migraines, and high blood pressure.

Biofeedback therapy helps a person to reduce tension, stress and also many other stress problems.

Researches have failed to find anything much about the mechanism of biofeedback. In this therapy, when you are stressed, a sensor is attached to your finger with the help of electrodes. It shows your heart rate, breath rate, blood pressure, body temperature, and muscle activity as a result of a monitor.

Biofeedback therapy is also useful in following:

- Schizophrenia
- Autism
- Eating disorders
- Anxiety
- Depression

Disadvantages of biofeedback therapy include:

- Chronic pain.
- Constipation.
- Irregular bowel syndrome.
- High blood pressure.
- Incontinence.
- Side effects of chemotherapy.
- Raynaud's disease. [20]

How can you avoid the weather?

The common and clear answer to the above question is that nobody can protect themselves from the hazards of the weather completely and this is scientifically proven that the weather triggers the migraine and headache.

According to research conducted to study the effect of weather on migraine sufferers, 62% of a person believed that weather triggered their migraine, though; in reality, only 51% were sensitive to the changes in weather.

As we already know that the change in the weather can trigger migraine and tension headaches. Following are some of the reasons that increase its chances:

- An abrupt decrease in the barometric pressure;
- Crucial weather change;
- High or low temperature with high humidity.

The storm, rain and the rise in temperature cause migraine and tension headache because the change in pressure leads to chemical and electrical changes in your brain which disturb the nerves and result in a migraine.

If you want to avert the migraine and chronic headache then use the weather forecast, which will help you to predict the migraine, and chronic headache attacks. You can always take prophylactic medication or measurements to prevent this headache.

Whenever there is unfavorable weather outside which might strike you, the best option is to remain indoor especially in air-conditioned rooms so that you can avoid the hazards of weather.

Be careful how you wash your hair!

According to the research in India, many migraine sufferers claim that they have a migraine attack when they wash their head while having a bath.

Additionally, the same research states that when some people dry their hair after hair wash, they tend to have a migraine and chronic headache attack.

Even this simple procedure can trigger the migraine attack. Next time keep this in your mind if you have never thought about it.

BEHAVIOURAL CHANGES TO REDUCE HEADACHES

Hair wash is a unique headache trigger. It may become better after taking preventive therapies. Some doctor suggests that taking Aleve and Ergo mar before hair wash averts the migraine attack after hair wash. [21]

9 Chapter Nine
DIFFERENT THERAPIES TO CURE HEADACHE

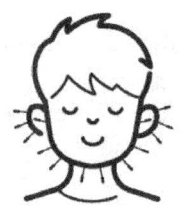

Hypnotherapy

Another beneficial therapy to reduce migraine and chronic headaches is hypnotherapy. In hypnotherapy, the experts practice hypnosis as a treatment. It is better to see a professional hypnotherapist to put in place hypnotherapy techniques if you find these techniques difficult to try on your own.

In this therapy, the experts use many techniques to transfer the person's focus away from the pain at the subconscious level towards a point where there is no pain.

The main task of the hypnotherapist is that you neglect the pain from which you are suffering and divert your focus toward the positive side of your life. This working of hypnosis helps headache sufferers to stop or reduce migraine and chronic pain. It is much better to hire a qualified hypnotherapist for better results.

Hypnotherapy is effective but only for those who have a severe headache. In severe headaches, it is difficult for a person to focus on any other thing because of the severity of pain. Hypnotherapy can help you to combat the pain and to decrease the duration as well.

Hypnotherapy also helps to reduce the intake of painkillers for headaches.

But the most important thing is that you must consult your doctor to find out whether your headache is associated with any co-morbidity or not before trying hypnotherapy. If there is any co-morbidity then treating that disease will help you in treating headaches. If there is no co-morbidity then you should go for hypnotherapy.

Benefits of Hypnotherapy are as follows:

- It will help you to reduce the pain of migraine and chronic headaches.
- It has no any kind of side-effects of your body and brain.

Hence, after reading enough about hypnotherapy, if you want to hire a therapist that helps you to change your focus at a subconscious level and forget about the headache, do give it a try. It will help you to lessen the severity of headache very swiftly. After attending one session, you will notice how simple it is to be hypnotized. With time, you can do it on your own and make it your routine to reduce the intensity of the headache.

However, many headache sufferers said that they feel comfortable working with a qualified professional hypnotherapist as compare to trying this technique by themselves at home.

If you are struggling to find any professional and highly qualified hypnotherapist that can help you to solve your problems. Do not worry just type hypnotherapists and your local area name on Google and find a qualified therapist near you. For instance, you live in Portland, Oregon and want to search a hypnotherapist near you then type hypnotherapist

How To Solve Migraine And Other Headaches

Portland and multiple searches will appear on your screen as shown in the following figure:

Here is the screenshot in which Google maps are showing the contact number and the address of the hypnotherapists as well. It helps you to make your first contact very easily.

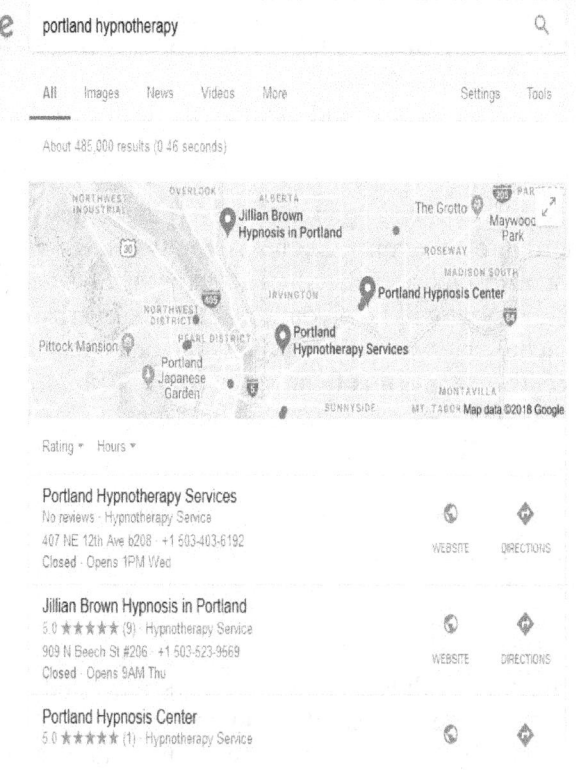

Furthermore, a standard Google search for 'online hypnotherapy' will throw up many sites where professional hypnotherapy advice and services are available online, so this is another option that you may like to consider:

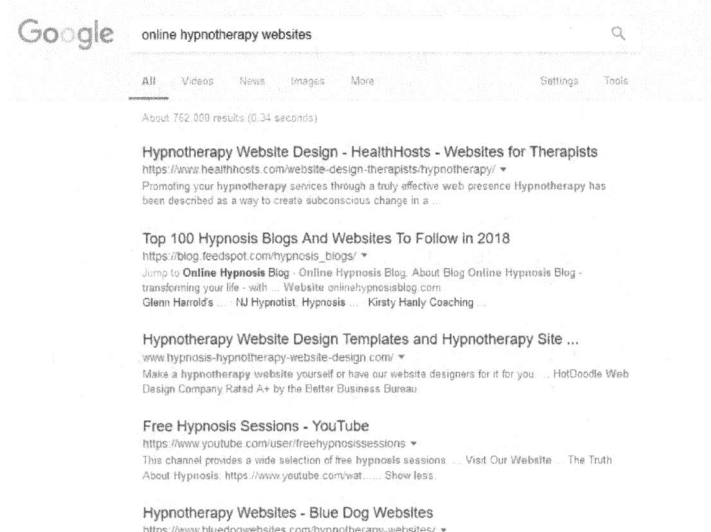

Moreover, there is another way to search on Google as well. For example, search for 'online hypnotherapy'. Multiple links of different sites will appear on the screen which not only provides online services but also give online professional hypnotherapy advice. The screenshot of this search is shown below:

Acupuncture or acupressure

Acupuncture is another method that several people use to reduce migraine or chronic headaches. It is quite similar to acupressure. The main functionality of both methods is to reduce the pain efficiently.

It is an old traditional Chinese method which is used as an alternative to medicine. In acupuncture, the needles are inserted in the body at different points to treat migraine, chronic headache, and many other medical disorders. The basic idea of acupuncture is that the channels or meridians through which the 'gi' or essential energy is streaming can be clogged. The whole procedure helps to reopen the channel or meridians that are blocked.

While, by putting needles at different acupuncture point at different depth levels, these blocked meridians or channels rehabilitate to their actual state:

Different Therapies To Cure Headache

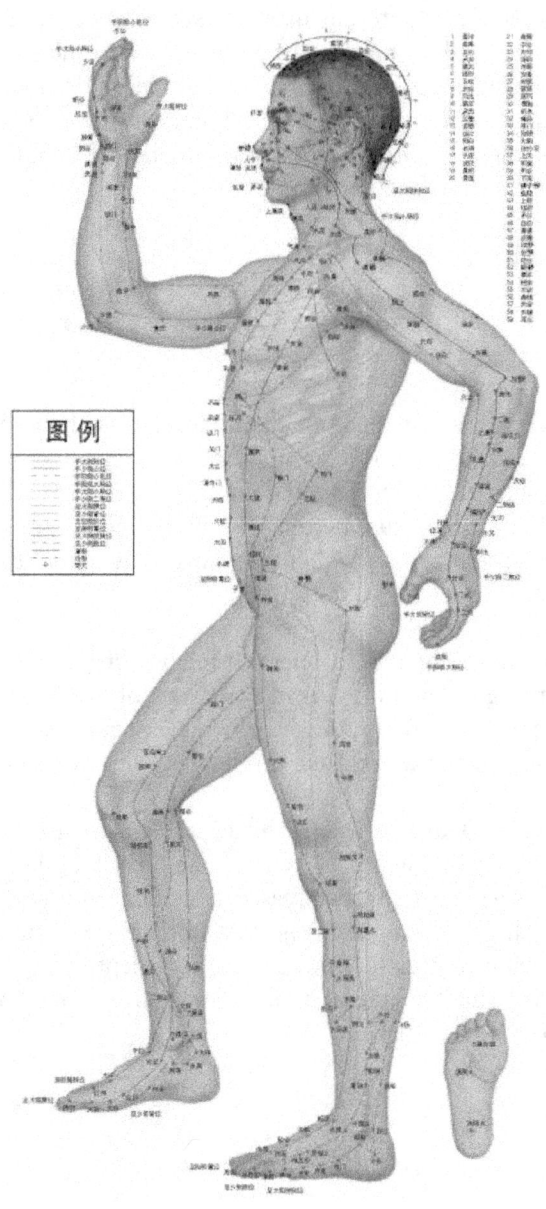

How To Solve Migraine And Other Headaches

In the West, acupuncture is usually used to treat different types of medical problems as well as migraine and chronic headaches. There is no clear-cut opinion in modern western medicine about the concept of meridians or channels and essential energy. Modern Western medicine still has a confused opinion about acupuncture.

But still, many western physicians trust acupuncture as a useful technique to treat several medical problems nowadays and many of the doctors have started to recommend their patients try acupuncture.

After the vast acceptance of acupuncture, it has become possible to seek a qualified and licensed practitioner in about every city in the West. If you are migraine or chronic sufferers, visit the acupuncture practitioner near your local area or search on Google about the nearby acupuncture specialist.

In acupuncture, the practitioner put the needles at the hé g point, through which they form a network of needles from thumb to palm. Usually, this hé g point is regarded as the most crucial point to treat the problems of head and face.

When the headache sufferers go and visit for their treatment, he is made to lie down in a comfortable position after that acupuncturist sterilizes the area on which he inserts the needles. Now the acupuncturist starts inserting the needles on the sterilized area to almost 3 to 5 mm depth until the patient feels the 'twinge' which indicates the 'hitting or reopening of the blockage'.

DIFFERENT THERAPIES TO CURE HEADACHE

After that 'twinge' feeling, the needle remains inserted for at least 15 to 20 minutes. During this time, many patients said that they feel satisfying tingling, a feeling of being relaxed and they also feel a noticeable reduction of pain in the head.

One of the most frequent misunderstandings about the acupuncture (which most of the time, draw many people away) is that it is very painful to insert the needle into the body. While, in reality, the needles that are used in acupuncture are multiple times finer than the hypodermic syringes. As compare to other syringes, it does not have a hollow center to inject the medicine. So, this perception is wrong that it is a painful process; it is very much painless as compared to most of the medical syringes.

As already mentioned, the insertion of needles is quite painless. It is the fear of the needle, which inhibits people from trying this procedure.

For those people, nowadays the acupuncturists use electro-acupuncture so that they can get the advantages of acupuncture. In electro-acupuncture, electronic probes are connected to the skin, they convey the electrical signal to 'unblock or reopen the meridians or channels) instead of using needles to unblock the meridians.

No doubt, most of the people believe that this way of treatment is more satisfying and less creepy than the traditional needle one. If you want this form of treatment, try to find any acupuncturists who have experience in electro-acupuncture.

How To Solve Migraine And Other Headaches

In acupuncture, applying pressure using thumbs, fingers, hands or even elbows is another way to unblock the meridians to the points where needles and electronic probes are usually used to restore the essential energy. All of these methods give the same results as they reduce the headache and many other medical problems.

The best thing about acupuncture is that once you have an idea of the location of the hé g then it is very easy for you to handle this specific area of your body on your own.

Now, whenever you are suffering from migraine or chronic headache, just massage the hé g point or the area between the thumb and palm. You will notice that it helps to reduce the severity of migraine and chronic headache. After that, you will understand the importance of that point for sure.

Some people share their experience that whenever that is suffering from migraine or chronic pain, they massage their temples, the back of the neck, and the sockets of their eyes and they realize that it reduces the migraine or chronic pain. This is another natural way of reducing the pain and the negative effects of headaches from the body.

Massage therapy for headaches...

Massage therapy is another convincing method, which is used to get rid of headaches. We can reduce the pain of any part of the body with the help of massage. Massage is the kneading and rubbing of the body tissues to get relaxation.

There are several types of massage therapies that are useful in making your body relaxed. In the USA only, according to a survey, there are more than 90,000 highly trained massage therapists. So, it is not hard to find a therapist that can give you a relaxing and pain-alleviating massage.

People after having a massage claim that it is very effective to reduce the pain from different parts of the body and consider it as a simple and brilliant way to reduce stress and headache.

Hence, if you are suffering from regular migraine or chronic headache and you are tired of medications and finding headache triggers, give massage therapy a try in such conditions.

Some massage center has also added aromatherapy in the regular massage. It is a fact that fusion of massage and aromatherapy can help in revitalizing your immune system as well.

The combination of the aromatherapy and massage is considered as the best combination because it stimulates and strengthens your immune system. It is also helpful in lowering the risk of having a migraine or chronic tension headaches

Other natural solutions for headaches

You should understand that every migraine or chronic headache sufferer find different methods effective for them. Every method is not useful to every sufferer.

In another way, every natural headache remedy or therapy that is available in this book is equally beneficial and safe to try. But still, you need to find out which one works best for you.

Unluckily, a negative aspect of this is every person needs to try several solutions before they find the best remedy for their migraine or chronic headache.

There are many different treatments that we have discussed in this book. All of these treatments are effective, beneficial and the best to lessen the migraine or chronic headaches according to many migraines or chronic headache sufferers. But make sure you understand that the first session of any remedy never gives you the required results.

Most of the headache sufferers used several remedies based on hit and trial before they find the perfect remedy for themselves that worked well for them. It needs lots of time and patience to get there. Different people get relief from different remedies. Even though all remedies are effective.

For the treatment of migraine or chronic headache, there are many herbal and natural remedies as well as traditional treatment written in this book. We recommend you to give them a try until and unless you find the best one.

10 Chapter Ten
HERBAL REMEDIES

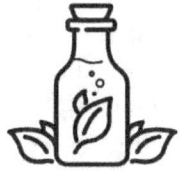

Feverfew (Tanacetum parthenium) is a herbal remedy that is used to reduce or lessen the intensity or frequency of migraine and headache. It is an ancient herbal method used to heal many different medical problems.

Though this herb was being used for many years, its effectiveness was still a topic of debate for experts. But now, current studies have proposed that about 6.25 mg of feverfew (Tanacetum parthenium) daily will help to avert the migraine attack and lessen the intensity of migraine or chronic headache.

After the observation of several years, it is also proven that coenzyme Q10 has a significant effect that prevents the migraine or chronic headache attack. In another experiment on some patients, it is shown that 100 mg dose of coenzyme Q10 for a few days prevent the migraine or chronic headache attack.

The best thing about these herbs is that they have shown side-effects to less than 1 percent of users. In a study spanning over several years, it was depicted that the side-effects of these herbs are only 1 percent more than the placebo drugs.

A few of the Vitamin B 'family' vitamins are also claimed to be useful in the prevention and treatment of migraine.

How To Solve Migraine And Other Headaches

Riboflavin is from the vitamin B2 family. In a placebo-controlled trial, it was observed that when the migraine or chronic headache sufferers used a dose of 400mg once a day regularly, it reduced the severity, duration of the frequency of migraine in sufferers.

In one experiment, a migraine sufferers' intake of vitamin B12 of 1mg dose once a day for three months proved that it decreases the intensity of migraines. More than 50% of the headache sufferers claim that having vitamin B12 in our daily reduces the migraine and chronic headache attack in the future.

Melatonin is another supplement that has beneficial effects that prevent migraine and chronic headaches attacks. It is a hormone, which is naturally present in several animals and plants like algae. If you want to buy it, you can easily find it online. Many websites are selling melatonin capsules. For this, you can do a search on Google like 'buy melatonin' or something like that.

Magnesium citrate is the main supplement, which is trusted to have the potential to lessen the intensity and frequency of migraine attacks. For example, in the placebo-controlled environment, some people who were having magnesium citrate in their daily routine diet had a remarkably lower rate of migraine than the people having the placebo in their diet...

REFERENCES

Some people who have taken 600mg of try magnesium dinitrate daily have claimed that they have 40% fewer migraine attacks in 9-12 weeks in an experiment, while the people under placebo group have 15.8% fewer migraine attacks.

Consequently, there are many natural remedies and nutritional supplements that can be used to stop or lessen the intensity and duration of migraine or chronic headache attacks.

Furthermore, we are going to discuss the final reason why you should prefer natural remedies instead of taking medicines and analgesics.

In reality, the intake of analgesics will make the migraine or the chronic headache pain pathetic, whether you believe it or not, painkillers extend the duration of migraine or chronic headache. On the contrary, if these same people stop taking any over-the-counter medication then they'll have a shortened period of migraine or chronic headaches.

Moreover, it may sound strange for you, but it is a fact that painkillers usually make your headache unpleasant, which is one of the main reasons for avoiding its usage.

CONCLUSION

As you have studied in this book, there are several different natural techniques from which you can get rid of migraine and chronic headaches thoroughly. It is good to use natural remedies to reduce your migraine or headache before moving towards the extremely damaging chemical-based medications.

As suggested earlier, people who have episodic tension headaches are so blessed that they only have a headache occasionally. These over-the-counter medications and painkillers may carry notable risks for teenagers and also for adults. But all of the natural treatments that are discussed in this book carry no any kind of harmful and serious side effects. So, your priority should be to try the natural remedies before going for the painkillers.

Briefly, if there is no other purpose of using it then it is always recommended, prefer using a natural treatment for any medical problem. It is always a better choice than using easily available over-the-counter medicines.

Certainly, all of the natural remedies that you came to know in this book are effective. As it is already suggested, not all remedies cure everyone's headache. A person who is suffering from a migraine or headache should try multiple solutions or remedies until unless they find the best one that cures their headache or migraine.

From now, no need to suffer the migraine pain that makes you miserable, and no need of having a pain killer to stop or reduce the intensity of migraine or headache attack.

Instead of taking a painkiller, try proper precautions and use natural treatments to heal the migraine or chronic headache. You can handle the entire issue naturally, without any type of side-effects on your brain and body.

REFERENCES

1. https://bit.ly/headache01
2. https://bit.ly/headache02
3. https://bit.ly/headache03
4. https://bit.ly/headache04
5. https://bit.ly/headache05
6. https://bit.ly/headache06
7. https://bit.ly/headache07
8. https://bit.ly/headache08
9. https://bit.ly/headache09
10. https://bit.ly/headache10
11. https://bit.ly/headache011
12. https://bit.ly/headache012
13. https://bit.ly/headache013
14. https://bit.ly/headache14
15. https://bit.ly/headache015
16. https://bit.ly/headache016
17. https://bit.ly/headache17
18. https://bit.ly/headache018
19. https://bit.ly/headache019
20. https://bit.ly/headache020
21. https://bit.ly/headache021

www.ingramcontent.com/pod-product-compliance
Lightning Source LLC
Chambersburg PA
CBHW071421220526
45469CB00004B/1373